MBIYA LUMBALA

A Manager's View of Public Health Services:

MBIYA LUMBALA

A Manager's View of Public Health Services:

The vital role played by vaccines against COVID-19

ScienciaScripts

Imprint

Any brand names and product names mentioned in this book are subject to trademark, brand or patent protection and are trademarks or registered trademarks of their respective holders. The use of brand names, product names, common names, trade names, product descriptions etc. even without a particular marking in this work is in no way to be construed to mean that such names may be regarded as unrestricted in respect of trademark and brand protection legislation and could thus be used by anyone.

Cover image: www.ingimage.com

This book is a translation from the original published under ISBN 978-620-6-71239-8.

Publisher:
Sciencia Scripts
is a trademark of
Dodo Books Indian Ocean Ltd. and OmniScriptum S.R.L publishing group

120 High Road, East Finchley, London, N2 9ED, United Kingdom
Str. Armeneasca 28/1, office 1, Chisinau MD-2012, Republic of Moldova, Europe
Printed at: see last page
ISBN: 978-620-8-13774-8

EPIGRAPH

"Fear is the first enemy of progress"

NSAMAN-O-L UTU Oscar (Phd)

INTRODUCTION

The year 2019 will forever be engraved in the history of humanity as the year that saw a catastrophe that plunged the whole world into mourning. It was in December 2019 that the world learned of the birth of an epidemic that originated in China and spread like lightning across the globe. From China, the epidemic reached Western Europe, then the American continent, and Africa was not spared.

Considered to be the epicentre of the epidemic, Chinese researchers will be deployed to combat this epidemic, which is spreading exponentially. Western researchers will not be kept on a leash. The death toll is in the thousands. The urgency imposed by the pandemic calls for emergency solutions.

In 2020, the first vaccines were developed on an experimental basis. While other parts of the world are rushing to get vaccinated, in Africa in general and the Democratic Republic of Congo in particular, mistrust of the vaccine is growing. Government communication has failed to take into account a number of factors that have led to mistrust among the people of Kinshasa. These include messages emanating from social networks and vaccination errors, which are contributing to the discouragement of the local population, creating mistrust and non-acceptability of the vaccine.

Faced with this unprecedented situation, we felt that it was possible to reverse the trend by creating the conditions required for Covid-19 vaccination to be accepted by the public. To this end, it would be useful to identify the key opinion leaders and resource people, and to involve young people in a wide-ranging awareness campaign.

1. **State of the question**

According to Matthieu TSHUNGU BAMESA, establishing the state of the question requires general knowledge of the subject through the literature. The appropriate formulation of hypotheses and the judicious choice of methods[5].

The state of the question in a scientific study is not simply a list of previous studies, but also a critical analysis of them. The aim is to identify the similarities and similarities with the current analyses under review. Such a critical analysis also enables us, as researchers, to identify the originality of our results, which we have achieved thanks to certain methods and techniques that we have used to achieve them.

These new results can therefore provide an objective assessment of the shortcomings of the previous stages, with a view to developing them further in the present and in the future. To put it more clearly, critical analysis helps to demonstrate the desirability of new developments or new conclusions[6].

No one can claim to contribute to the development of scientific knowledge in a given field without conducting a literature review. This intellectual exercise enables us to show the particularity of our study in

---

[5] MBIYA LUMBALA,E. :Management public pour l'efficacité des services publics de l'Etat dans la ville province de Kinshasa de 2006-2019,Mémoire de DEA, Fac. Management et Sciences économiques. CEPROMAD,2018

[6] TSHUNGU BAMESA, M., *Du travail scientifique à ¡'Université,* ed. Africa, Lubumbashi, 2017, p.16.

relation to a number of previous works that have tackled more or less the same theme. It is to visit previous studies and propose new avenues for solutions to the problems surrounding man in society.

Secondly, research cannot be organised from scratch; it can only be undertaken through a critical evaluation of prior knowledge. These may appear to the researcher in various forms: events or concrete data, but also ideas, concepts, explanations or interpretations directly or indirectly concerning his study. This critical approach is fundamental; it is a prerequisite for the research, and then determines the various stages.

In addition, among the previous studies that have dealt with the same subject, a number of authors have taken into account the known data on the COVID 19 vaccine, the integration of strategic and operational management as a relevant immunisation planning tool in relation to the experiences of similar immunisation campaigns.

1.1. Compared to COVID 19 vaccines

A meta-analysis of the potential acceptability of the COVID-19 vaccine found that 71.5% of people worldwide would be very or fairly likely to take the vaccine against COVID-19. However, the rate of acceptance varies considerably from one country to another. The highest acceptance rates in the world were observed in Ecuador (97.0%), Malaysia (94.3%) and Indonesia (93.3%). The lowest acceptance rates for the

COVID-19 vaccine were observed in Kuwait (23.6%) and Jordan (28.4%).

In Africa, a study carried out in Uganda showed an acceptance rate for the COVID-19 vaccine of 53%, and in Nigeria the rate was 51.1%. In the DRC, vaccination began on 19 April 2021, and to date 15,404 people have already been vaccinated in Kinshasa. Vaccination activities are slow in Kinshasa and throughout the country. Vaccination programmes only succeed when acceptance and coverage rates are high.

To do this, it is essential to understand the level of acceptance of the COVID-19 vaccine in the DRC and the factors associated with its rejection, particularly in Kinshasa, which is the province most affected by this pandemic, accounting for more than 70% of cases nationwide. To achieve herd immunity, with an R0 of 3, a minimum of 67% of the population of Kinshasa must be vaccinated. The Kinshasa School of Public Health assessed the knowledge, attitudes and practices of the population in four communes of the city of Kinshasa in 2020. It would be important to know the acceptability of the covid 19 vaccine in the community, the factors associated with resistance to the covid 19 vaccine, and to assess the extent to which strategic and operational management have been taken into account in measures to combat covid 19 in order to rectify the situation in the provincial city.

1.2. In relation to vaccination errors

According to the Vaccine Adverse Reporting System (VAERS) report published in the United States for the period from 2000 to 2013, out of a total of 311,185 MAPI cases, 20,585 or 7% were linked to vaccination errors. Of these vaccination errors, 5,504, or 25%, had an adverse health effect, compared with 15,381, or 75%, which did not. According to the same report, serious IPD accounted for 407, or 8%.

2. In relation to vaccination in general

The implementation of safe and practical injection policies in the Expanded Programme on Immunisation (EPI) and numerous Supplementary Immunisation Activities (SIAs) over the past two decades may also have contributed to the overall reduction in the programme error rate([7]).

Five questions were used to measure the perception of the risk of contracting COVID 19: the risk of contracting the disease; the fear of contracting the disease; the perception of the curability of the disease and the effectiveness of prevention measures; and the acceptability of prevention measures by the community. As for attitudes, two questions were asked to measure the level of stigmatisation against COVID 19. A

---

total score was calculated.

3. **Prevention practices and challenges encountered in implementing these prevention measures**

Preventive practices against COVID 19 were measured by respondents' self-declaration. The items were taken from a similar survey conducted in Iran (13) and from the barrier measures recommended by the WHO and the DRC Ministry of Health. The following items were sought: restriction of movement (five questions); prevention practices during coughing (one question); social distancing (one question); hand hygiene (one question); use of a social mask (one question); avoidance of touching the face with unwashed hands (one question); avoidance of hand-waving or kissing (one question); discussion of COVID 19 prevention with family or friends (one question).

4. **Acceptability of the vaccine**

We asked participants if they would be willing to receive a vaccine to protect themselves against the coronavirus, if a vaccine were made available in the country. This variable was collected on a nominal scale (binary qualitative) coded 0 if the participant expressed willingness to be vaccinated and 1 in the case of refusal.

5. **Reason for non-acceptance of the vaccine**

For participants who had not expressed a wish to receive the vaccine, additional questions were asked to understand the reasons for this refusal.

World Health Organization. Immunization, vaccines and biological La Corona Virus Disease 19 (COVID-19) which believes that COVID-19 is a pandemic that began on December 31, 2019 in China in the city of Wuhan.[8]

Eduard B, Batson A. Using believes that in Africa, in a study conducted in Uganda, a 53% acceptance rate of the COVID-19 vaccine was observed[9] .

WHO and UNICEF[10] believe that the current COVID-19 pandemic has had serious repercussions on the health, security and economy of the continent, and the DRC has not been spared.

2. Issues

The subject of any scientific work is certainly a problem that is fundamentally posed in terms of the given social realities and which requires the formulation of appropriate solutions. The problem thus becomes "a set of questions that the researcher asks himself about his research subject. In short, it is the author's major concern. The problematic is the materialization of a researcher's concern, expressed in the questions

---

[8] World Health Organization. Immunization, vaccines and biological. Geneva, consulted on 16 June 2015

[9] Eduard B, Batson A. Using immunization coverage rates for monitoring health sector performance: Measurement and interpretation issues. Human development network, The World Bank; Washington, 2004.

[10] WHO, UNICEF, Global Immunization: Strategic Vision 2006-2015, Geneva, 2006, p. 82.

he or she asks about his or her research subject.

Despite the severity of the pandemic and the availability of the vaccine, the Congolese population in general and Kinshasa in particular refused to be vaccinated. Vaccination has been one of the great successes of public health. It has saved the lives of millions of children and given millions of others the prospect of a longer life in better health, as well as better opportunities to learn, read and write, and to play and move around freely without suffering[11] .

Nevertheless, vaccine-preventable diseases remain a major cause of morbidity and mortality worldwide. There are currently vaccines against more than 25 infectious diseases, and the number of vaccines is constantly increasing, as in the case of the vaccines against COVID 19.

However, despite its protective effect, resistance to vaccination is still gaining ground. Vaccines can directly or indirectly cause adverse events, the occurrence of which must be monitored and managed to promote the use of health services and manage resistance. It is expected that the administration of a WHO prequalified vaccine on a routine or campaign basis will not generate serious MAPI beyond acceptable thresholds (< 1 to 3/1000000). Serious IPD highlights

---

[11] (7)Nelson Mandela
2002, president - Vaccine Fund Board

The need for hospitalisation or ;

- The need for extended hospitalisation or ;

- Life-threatening or ;

- Death or ;

- Persistent disability or ;

- The effect on the design product.

The opposite of "serious" is "non-serious". This category includes mild fever ($<$ or $= 38°C$), headache, digestive problems, pain and redness at the injection site.

The administration of a new vaccine, such as the one against COVID 19, by health workers who are insufficiently trained for the purpose, less attentive to storage, transport and handling conditions, and who are unsupervised or inadequately supervised, is conducive to avoidable PAD in vaccinated patients. It is this perception as a whole that accentuates the fear of vaccines.

IPMs often cause great concern in the communities concerned, who end up abandoning vaccination services, and very often the staff who are supposed to be behind these IPMs flee the services or are brought before the courts. Parents, guardians or the victims themselves, who are initially in apparently good health, find it hard to understand why they should suffer, rightly or wrongly, the adverse effects of vaccines because they have accepted a vaccine for which assurances of safety, efficacy and tolerance have been widely publicised.

In the current era, it is no secret that vaccination remains a solution to the COVID-19 health crisis, which constitutes a major collective public health issue. This leads us to the following research problem:

What factors explain the population's refusal of the Covid-19 vaccine in the provincial city of Kinshasa?

3. Assumptions

On the basis of the research question posed above, the hypotheses are as follows:

- the absence of strategic and operational management is not conducive to the implementation of prevention-related activities;

- the population's resistance to vaccination is directly linked to the occurrence of IBD;

- the sidelining of community leaders at various levels has accentuated the population's rejection of vaccines;

* social networks have had a major impact on the official channels for raising public awareness of vaccines

3.1. Objectives

Two categories of objectives are assigned to this work, namely general and specific.

3.2 **General objective**

The aim is to contribute to the fight against COVID 19, with a view to bringing the pandemic to an end.

3.3 **Specific objectives**

The specific objectives are set out below:

> Determine the frequency of people refusing vaccines according to socio-economic background ;

> Identify the factors associated with this resistance in the provincial city of Kinshasa;

> Assess the extent to which strategic and operational management are taken into account in measures to combat COVID 19 ;

> Formulate suggestions at different levels to rectify the situation ;

The low uptake of Covid-19 vaccination by the population of the city and province of Kinshasa is due to the population's resistance to vaccination as a result of the fear of post-vaccination adverse events (MAPI) widely disseminated on social networks.

❖ The country's authorities did not get vaccinated, health workers who were supposed to set an example refused to be vaccinated, and so on.

❖ The failure of the campaign meant that planning was carried out through the RIA, which led to the development of the PNDV.

❖ Here are some of the challenges that were addressed during an intra-action review organised by the Ministry of Public Health in August 2021:

❖ Late response to the half-hearted information on vaccination;

❖ Weak mobilisation of APAs and influencers at all levels in favour of vaccination against COVID-19 ;

❖ Weak implementation of interpersonal communication, local mobilisation (CODESA, CAC/ReCo) ;

❖ Weak support for the provincial level from the central level (supervision of communication activities by the central level);

4. Announcement of the methodological approach

Methodology" can be explained as a branch of epistemology that studies research methods and techniques. The drafting of any scientific work inevitably involves a methodological perspective, likely to serve as a heuristic instrument for interrogating reality. This study is no exception to this scientific requirement"[12] . The second chapter is devoted to the methodological approach.

5. Choice and interest of subject

---

[12]   GRAWITZ M and PINTO R.,

This dissertation was designed to obtain the Diplôme d'Etude Approfondi en Management et Sciences Economiques, Orientation Management des Santés Publiques at the University of CEPROMAD. Its choice was dictated by professional considerations. In view of the topicality of this subject, which remains at the centre of institutional and academic reflection on resistance to vaccination against COVID-19 and the lack of integration of management as a strategy in the public health system in the city of Kinshasa.

With regard to its originality and interest, we have integrated into this analysis a strategic and operational management approach in the public health system capable of combating this resistance to vaccination in the area under study. The aim is to gain a managerial perspective. This leads us to the following research question:

- Why is the population of the provincial city of Kinshasa refusing the Covid-19 vaccine?

6. **Work delimitation**

The complexity of social phenomena requires any scientific work to be delimited in time and space. Delimiting the work is both an indispensable requirement and a guarantee of the circumscription necessary for its proper understanding. This work is no exception to this requirement.

In terms of time, this study covers the period from March 2020 to

June 2021. This delimitation is no accident. The first boundary marks the start of the Covid-19 pandemic in the Democratic Republic of Congo in general, and in Kinshasa in particular, with the detection of the first case. The second boundary coincides with the mobilisation of the response team, which is determined to reduce the pandemic and raise public awareness of the importance of vaccination.

7. The work of our partners

In addition to the general introduction and conclusion, this work is divided into three chapters. The first chapter comprises two sections: the first outlines the conceptual framework. The second sets out the theoretical framework. The first section highlights the concepts of resistance, vaccination, Covid 19, strategic and operational management and the health system. The second section looks at the theoretical framework for work based on Communication for Social Change.

The second chapter presents the methodological approach to the work. The third chapter presents, analyses, interprets and discusses the results. The aim is to explain the factors that explain resistance to vaccination against Covid 19. This chapter suggests the integration of strategic and operational management in the healthcare system to reduce resistance to vaccination against the COVID-19 pandemic.

CHAPTER I: GENERAL THEORETICAL CONSIDERATIONS

The first section examines the main concepts used in this work. These are the concepts of Covid-19, strategic and operational management, resistance, the health system and immunisation. The second section sets out the theoretical framework for this work, which is based on behaviour change communication theory.

Section I. Conceptual framework

1.1. Covid-19

The aim here is to trace the development of the pandemic and its successive waves.

1.1.1. Evolution of the pandemic

Corona Virus Disease 19 (COVID-19) is a pandemic that began on 31 December 2019 in China in the city of Wuhan, Hubei province. It has been declared a public health emergency of international concern by the World Health Organization (WHO)[13] . As of Sunday 13 June 2021, the covid-19 virus has affected 175,488,504 (+36,228) confirmed cases and caused a total of 3,784,087 (+762) deaths worldwide. In Africa, there have been more than 2,999,152 confirmed cases and more than 76,113 deaths. The burden of COVID-19 is still increasing, especially in Europe and the Americas. As of 13 June 2021, the Democratic Republic of Congo (DRC)

---

[13] WHO, UNICEF. Global Immunization: Strategic Vision 2006 - 2015. Geneva. 2006; p. 82.

has reported 35,668 confirmed cases, including 25,559 in Kinshasa, and 846 deaths[14] .

The current COVID-19 pandemic has had serious repercussions for health, security and the economy across the continent, and the DRC has not been spared.

In April 2020, the IMF (International Monetary Fund) revised its 2020 global economic growth forecasts, projecting a 3% contraction in the world economy. This recession is far more serious than the 2008-2009 financial crisis.

I.1.2. Treatment of the pandemic

In a WHO report[15] , she believes that to date there is no specific treatment for COVID-19, which makes preventive measures such as wearing masks, hand washing and social distancing one of the main options for curbing the pandemic. However, these have a considerable impact on the psychosocial well-being of the population. In early November 2020, the first results of the major phase 3 COVID-19 vaccine trials were announced. More than 30 candidate vaccines have been or are currently being evaluated in advanced clinical trials. Safety and efficacy data of up to 95% have been

---

[14] WHO AFRO. Guidelines for the evaluation of Supplementary Measles Immunization Activities, revised January 2006.

[15] WHO, op. cit,

reported[16] .

Many countries around the world have begun to vaccinate their populations with vaccines that have been shown to be effective, and many others are preparing to do so. A vaccine is a therapy consisting of stimulating an individual's immune system so as to obtain a specific response from the body against a given antigen, whether viral, bacterial, cellular or even molecular. An effective vaccine against the coronavirus will help save lives and ensure a gradual return to "normal" life on a global scale. Optimal vaccination of the population could rapidly and effectively reduce the burden of the pandemic.

A meta-analysis of the potential acceptability of the COVID-19 vaccine found that 71.5% of people worldwide would be very or fairly likely to take the vaccine against COVID-19. However, the rate of acceptance varies considerably from one country to another. The highest acceptance rates in the world were observed in Ecuador (97.0%), Malaysia (94.3%) and Indonesia (93.3%). And the lowest acceptance rates for the COVID-19 vaccine were observed in Kuwait (23.6%) and Jordan (28.4%).

In Africa, a study carried out in Uganda showed an acceptance rate for the COVID-19 vaccine of 53%, while in Nigeria the rate was 51.1%.

---

[16] World Health Organization. Global Advisory Committee on Vaccine Safety, 9-10 June 2005. Weekly Epidemiological Record, 2005, 80:242-247.

Vaccination in the DRC began on 19 April 2021, and to date 15,404 people have already been vaccinated in Kinshasa. Vaccination activities are slow in the city of Kinshasa and throughout the country in general. Vaccination programmes only succeed when acceptance and coverage rates are high. To achieve this, it is essential to understand the level of acceptance of the COVID-19 vaccine in the DRC, as well as the factors associated with its rejection, particularly in Kinshasa, which is the province most affected by this pandemic, accounting for more than 70% of cases nationwide. To achieve herd immunity, a minimum of 67% of the population of Kinshasa needs to be vaccinated[17] .

I.1.3. Different waves of the pandemic

After the first and second waves of the pandemic, since May 2021 the country has been faced with a third wave of the COVID-19 pandemic, the epidemiology of which is evolving rapidly throughout the world and is accompanied by the emergence of new variants. As of 11 July 2021, the DRC was the 17th most affected country in the WHO-AFRO region, with a total of 44,333 confirmed cases, and the 18th country with the most deaths (984), with a case-fatality rate of 2.2%. A total of 25 (96.2%) of the country's 26 provinces are affected. In cumulative terms since the start of the epidemic, the province of Kinshasa is the epicentre of COVID-19 (71.5%), followed by the provinces of Nord-Kivu (8.2%), Kongo central

WHO, UNICEF. COVID-19: strategic vision 2006 - 2015. Geneva. 2006; p. 82.

(5.6%), Haut Katanga (5.2%), Lualaba (2.6%) and Sud-Kivu (2.2%).

To tackle this pandemic, in addition to the other control measures in place, the global community is working to develop new vaccines and make them available. It is within this framework that the COVAX initiative has been set up, with the aim of guaranteeing equitable access to vaccines for all countries. It is within this framework that the country has been supplied with vaccine (1,766,000 doses of AZD1222) since 02 March 2021.

Since 19 April 2021, the DRC has been gradually introducing the COVID-19 vaccine in the 6 most affected provinces, starting in the provincial city of Kinshasa. The extension of this vaccination has been extended to other provinces in the country, taking into account the epidemiological evolution of the pandemic and the level of preparations in each province. The roll-out of this vaccination against Covid-19 has been marked by slowness and low uptake by the beneficiary populations, which has led to the redeployment of most of the vaccine doses to other countries to avoid them expiring.

In the meantime, the country has embarked on the fight without a strategic or operational management process. It was the population's resistance at the end of the 1ère vaccination campaign that prompted the authorities of the Ministry of Public Health, Prevention and Hygiene, at various levels and with the support of partners, to plan for the implementation of the National Vaccine and Immunisation Deployment Plan, with the involvement of the population through the various community-based bodies.

I.2. Strategic and Operational Management

I.2.1. Management

The term management is commonly used these days, but not always in a coherent way, as the concept is often very approximate in everyday practice.

According to Oscar NSAMAN-O-LUNTU, management is integrated into his paradigm of "an elephant surrounded by twenty blind men "[14] . In other words, each blind man (the elephant) will define management according to the part affected.[18] [19] [20] [21]

According to Henry Mintzeberg, management is "a process by which those who have formal responsibility for all or part of an organisation attempt to direct it, or at least to guide it in its activities "[16].

For KOOTZ and O'donnell, management is "far from having a standardised meaning, although it is generally agreed that the word refers to the performance of tasks by people "[17].

Other authors, such as Peter Drucker, believe that management is

---

(14)   Oscar NSAMAN-O-LUTU and Godé ATSHWEL, *Comprendre le management, Principes, Outils, Cultures et Contingence,* Kinshasa, Ed. CAPM, 2007.
(15)   MORSON, M.A., *Dictionnaire du Management stratégique,* Paris, Ed. Belin sup, 2000, RPS-8.
19
20
21

"essentially a form of corporate governance in which the processes of transformation in which the company communicates with its market are closely coordinated and regular at the level of leadership and management. They transform information into action and ensure the availability of resources "[18].

We consider management to be the combination of four axes: Culture, Contingency, Principle and Tools. Finally, management means a rational decision-making process that prevents the fallout from that decision from being passed on to the decision-makers.

I.2.2. Strategic management

a. Definition

Strategic management concerns the medium and long term (> 2 years) and is the sole responsibility of general management. Management must have a vision to ensure the future of the organisation. Management defines the direction and objectives of the organisation and the most appropriate structure for the organisation. Senior management sets the objectives and chooses the means of achieving them, taking into account the various constraints facing the organisation.

b. Strategic decisions

A strategic decision commits the organisation over the long term.

This type of decision may or may not ensure the future of the organisation. It is a one-off decision that cannot be reversed, and cannot be programmed because it is unpredictable and complex. General management takes this type of decision, but the consequences of these decisions affect everyone in the organisation.

Ultimately, we believe with NSAMAN that strategic management in the context of our subject is nothing other than the different visions or programmes of the WHO or the political authorities had to hang on to in order to get the Covid-19 vaccine accepted.

I.2.3. Operational management

a. Definition

- Operational management has two main functions: Mobilising and allocating resources to achieve the objectives set by strategic management;
- To coordinate the actions of the various members of the organisation.

Operational management operates in three areas: organisational, technical and human.

b. Operational decisions

The time horizon for operational decisions is the short term. This type of decision does not, a priori, entail any risk for the survival of the organisation. It is a frequent decision, not very complex and therefore programmable. An operational decision can be taken by all the staff in the organisation, even if operational management is often entrusted to the management staff.

3. Relevance of the strategic/operational separation

a. Taylorian concept of separation

With the scientific organisation of work, F.W. Taylor sought to rationalise work by separating design from execution.

For him, strategic management is the brain of the organisation and operational management is the arms of the organisation. This vision has been called into question by modern organisations.

b. Questioning the separation

Strategic management sets the course for operational management. Operational managers must adapt to strategic decisions, but they do not always have the skills to implement these strategic decisions effectively. This skill constraint often takes second place to financial, technological and commercial constraints. The distinction between strategic and operational management is not always clear.

Let's take the example of prisoners who escape from a prison. Does this incident fall under the operational heading, with a lack of supervision by prison guards, or does it fall under the strategic heading, with a prison lacking security due to a lack of funding? The contemporary conception of the organisation blurs the separation between the strategic and the operational.

The essentials

Strategic management guides the organisation over the long term to ensure its future.

Operational management develops a short-term action plan to achieve the objectives set by strategic management.

The contemporary conception of the organisation blurs the separation between the strategic[22] and the operational.

	Strategic decisions	Operational decisions
Hierarchical level at which the decision is taken	General Management	Management staff
Time horizon	Long-term (> 2 years)	Short term (< 2 years)
Degree of repetitiveness	Single decision not programmable because not	Frequent, uncomplicated decisions
	predictable and complex	programmable

---

[22] NSAMAN-O-LUTU opcit

Table 1: Elements of strategic and operational management Source

Ultimately, we believe that strategic management is nothing more than the application of the vision or programmes adopted by the authority.

1.1.3. Resistance

LE VILAIN believes that the concept of *resistance only appeared in literature towards* the end of the 13th century[e] . It means "the quality by which one body resists the action of another body "[20].

Resistance is the "force that opposes or cancels out the effect of another force" ([21] hence 1883 *electrical resistance* "ratio of the power lost in a circuit in the form of heat or radiation to the square of the intensity of the instantaneous conduction current". Conductor designed to release a specific thermal power "quality of what resists, resistant character "[22]. ORESME thinks that in a meal, *pièce de* **résistance**, pièce considérable, où il y a beaucoup à manger).

CHRISTINE DE PISAN goes on to say that "resistance is the action of defending oneself with weapons, of opposing by force a person or group that uses force or physical coercion".[*21 22 23 24 25 26]

MAHIEU LE VILAIN, *Metheores d'Aristote,* ed. R. Edgren, p. 38, lines 30 and 31
[24] (JACQUEZ, *Dict. d'électr. et de magnét. ,*); 1883, p. 172,SN
[25] (ORESME, *Ethiques,* ed. A. D. Menut, VII, 12, f° 144c, p. 387); 1798 *(Ac.:*
[26] (CHRISTINE DE PISAN, *Livre de Charles V,* ed. S. Solente, t. 1, p. 130);

In the context of this study, the concept of resistance is used as a synonym for failure, to show the extent to which the population of Kinshasa has not embraced the Covid-19 vaccination programme.

1.1.4. Health system

Zhou P., Yang X.L., and Wang X.G. believe that the concept of "healthcare system" brings together "all the organisations, institutions and resources involved in healthcare and which provide formal care (doctors, clinics, hospitals and pharmacies), informal care (traditional healers, community workers) and other services, such as research".

But beyond that, a health system comprises a great many other elements - everything that helps to promote or protect health "[24].

A healthcare system describes the organisational and strategic resources put in place by country, geographical area or community entity to ensure continuity and quality of healthcare services.

The study of a health system enables us to describe, by jurisdiction, the nature and operation of medical and social care, the financing and management of health-related expenditure, the means of combating, preventing or promoting health implemented as part of health policies, the deployment and training of human resources and the scientific research resources put in place.

I.1.5. Vaccination

According to Larousse, vaccination means "administration of a vaccine with the effect of conferring active immunity, specific to a disease, making the organism resistant to this disease "[25].

According to the World Health Organisation (WHO), vaccination is "a simple, safe and effective way of protecting yourself from dangerous diseases, before you come into contact with them. It uses the body's natural defences to create resistance to specific infections and strengthen the immune system" [26]. In other words, vaccines stimulate the immune system to create antibodies, in the same way as if it were exposed to the disease. But because vaccines only contain killed or attenuated forms of germs, viruses or bacteria, they do not cause disease and do not expose the subject to the risk of complications. [***27 28 29]

So to speak, most vaccines are administered by injection, but some are taken orally or by nasal spray. However, it's worth asking what a vaccine actually consists of.

A vaccine consists of "injecting an infectious agent (virus or bacteria) into the body in a harmless form that stimulates the body's immune response. As the immune system has a form of memory, subsequent

---

[24] Zhou P., Yang X.L., Wang X.G., Hu B., Zhang L., Zhang W. A pneumonia outbreak associated with a new coronavirus of probable bat origin. *Nature.* 2020;579(7798):270-273
[25]
[26] WHO

exposure to the infectious agent will trigger a rapid and therefore more effective response. The agent is recognised by one or more specific molecules and constitutes the antigen"[30] . The immune system responds by producing antibodies specifically directed against it and manufactured by memory cells (B and T lymphocytes). A vaccine is therefore specific to a disease.

---

[30] https://www.futura-sciences.com, accessed on 27 August 2021 at 15:25.

Section II. Theoretical framework

The second section sets out the theoretical framework for the study. All scientific research is rooted in a theoretical framework. It is the foundation that justifies the raison d'être of the research. This work is in line with this logic.

1.2.1. Relevance of the theoretical framework

It goes without saying that, in order to consolidate the theoretical basis of a scientific study, the researcher must be able to validate his choice of concepts and consolidate his problematic and hypotheses by inserting them into a proven current of thought. Following this scientific approach, this work cannot escape this requirement.

1.2.2. Communication Theory for Social Behaviour Change

As part of this study into resistance to vaccination against covid-19 and the lack of integration between strategic and operational management, we used Communication for Social and Behavioural Change. This theory of change aims to bring greater clarity and quality to the process of designing and implementing programmes, by applying a simple and flexible method.

Communication for social and behavioural change is an approach that promotes and facilitates changes in knowledge, attitudes, norms, beliefs and behaviours (CAC/BCC). The acronyms BCC and SBCC are often used interchangeably. They both refer to a series of activities and strategies that promote healthy behaviour. The word "social" has been added to the BCC concept to indicate that to improve health outcomes, it is necessary to support wider social change.

A strategic approach to communication for social and behaviour change follows a systematic process for analysing a problem to identify the key barriers and motivators for change, and then designing and implementing a comprehensive set of interventions to support and encourage positive behaviours. A communication strategy guides CCC campaigns and interventions, ensuring that communication objectives are defined, target audiences identified and consistent messages determined for all materials and activities. Effective SCCC programmes use different communication channels to reach their targets.

There are various models and frameworks available to guide the planning of SCCC programmes. Most share the same basic principles. The process is a widely used model for planning an intervention or campaign: it provides a step-by-step guide from exploring a briefly defined behaviour change concept to developing a strategic and participatory programme that is grounded in theory and has a measurable impact. To achieve this, five steps need to be integrated into the analysis process. These include analysis, strategic design, development and pre-testing, implementation and monitoring, and evaluation and evolution.

Three cross-cutting concepts are integrated into the behaviour change process. Their integration ensures greater effectiveness of Communication for Social Behaviour Change approaches, in this case the theory of communication for social behaviour change, stakeholder participation and ongoing capacity building.

The examples below clearly show that it is possible to achieve good communication for behaviour change when there is follow-up and when young people are involved.

So you've probably seen examples of SCCC activities in your town, for example :

A mass media campaign promoting the use of condoms to prevent HIV and other STIs through advertisements in public services and/or soap operas broadcast on radio or television.

A theatre group performing a play about gender-based violence for a community and holding a discussion afterwards.

A radio programme that answers listeners' questions about family planning.

A school programme that encourages pupils to wait before having sex for the first time.

A short message service (SMS) or helpline providing information on family planning or HIV. Reaching young people with SCCC programmes in urban areas has specific advantages and disadvantages.

An overarching theory of change should be developed for the UNDAF to help explain the outcome areas prioritised by the UN system and to promote gender equality in the event that a separate outcome is not dedicated to it. In addition, theories of change can be developed for each outcome area as a basis for identifying and explaining the UNDAF outputs in the joint work plans of the outcome groups. This methodology recommends three core principles and four sequential steps for developing a theory of change.

A) The theory of change should be developed in a consultative manner to take into account the understanding of all stakeholders;

B) It should be based on sound evidence, and tested and revised on the basis of that evidence at all stages; and

C) It should be based on continuous learning and improvement, from the design to the closure of programmes.

Behaviour change communication has many advantages and few disadvantages, which we summarise here.

1.2.3. Advantages, disadvantages of the theory and links with the object of study

The advantages enjoyed by teenagers in urban areas include, for example, greater access to different media and technological possibilities, and the healthcare services available to them are more numerous and varied. The high population density also means that many teenagers can be affected at the same time.

Now that we've talked about the advantages, there's no shortage of disadvantages. Urban teenagers tend to be more mobile, which means it's difficult to reach the same teenager several times with your message. Slums make it difficult to get the message across, and the lack of traditional family structures for many urban teenagers means that they may not have the support within the home to reinforce messages about healthy behaviour.

CHAPTER II: METHODOLOGICAL APPROACH TO THE WORK

The second chapter focuses on the methodological path that led to the expected results. Any epistemological approach requires methods and techniques. Scientific research always requires the choice of a methodological approach to guide data analysis and interpretation. This is why scientific work requires a rational approach to arrive at scientific knowledge or the truth.

2.1. Method

Etymologically, the word "method" comes from the Greek meaning path or route to follow to reach the goal. PINTO and GRAWITZ believe that method is the set of intellectual operations, norms and rules by which the researcher gathers, classifies and explains facts in order to build up scientific knowledge[31] . They define method as the set of intellectual operations by which a discipline seeks to attain the truths it pursues, verifies them and demonstrates them[32] .

2.2. Study framework[33]

The study took place in the provincial city of Kinshasa. The capital

---

[31] PINTO, R. and GRAWITZ, M., *Méthode des sciences sociales,* Paris, 2ème éd. Dalloz, 1976, p.2.
[20] Idem, p.13.
[33] This presentation is taken from Institut National de Statistique, *Profil de la ville de Kinshasa,* November 2015.

of the Democratic Republic of Congo, it is also the seat of the country's political institutions. Located in the west of the country, the city covers an area of at least 10,000 km² (or 9,965 km²). In 2015, the National Institute of Statistics estimated the population of this city-province at around 11.6 million inhabitantsl , or 13.6% of the national population (85.026 million). Population density is very high (averaging over 1,000 inhabitants/km²) compared with the national average (36 inhabitants/km²). The province's soil is mainly sandy and of little use for farming. As a result, there is no specific agricultural product that characterises this province, which is mainly supplied with agricultural products from Kongo Central, Bandundu and Equateur.

2.3. Type of study

This is a cross-sectional descriptive study with an analytical focus.

2.4. Study period

This study covers the period from March 2020 to June 2021. This delimitation is not random. The first boundary marks the start of the Covid-19 pandemic in the Democratic Republic of Congo in general, and in Kinshasa in particular, with the detection of the first case. The second boundary coincides with the mobilisation of the response team, which is determined to reduce the pandemic and raise public awareness of the importance of vaccination.

2.5. Study population

The study population consisted of the inhabitants of the provincial city of Kinshasa, in the 19 Health Zones.

2.5.1. Sample size

The sample size description was calculated as follows:

* Compared to Active surveillance

Calculating the sample size :

$$n = z^2 \times \frac{P \times Q}{d^2}$$

Z = 1.96 for a 95% confidence level

Q =1-p

d= tolerated margin of error or degree of precision sought

P from MAPI = estimate of the prevalence sought (i.e. a prevalence

of 50%, which gives a maximum sample size)

- P= 0.5 (prevalence = 50%)

- Q = 1 - P = 0.5

- z = 1,96 = 2

$$n = \frac{(1{,}96)^2 \times 0{,}5 \times 0{,}5}{(0{,}05)^2} = \frac{3{,}8416 \times 0{,}25}{0{,}0025} = 384{,}16 \cong 384$$

But if we round the value of z to 2,

$$n = \frac{4 \times 0,25}{0,0025} = 400$$

We increased this sample to 627 respondents in order to research the components of resistance factors.

2.5.2 Sampling

Sampling was carried out at several levels:

First level: Selection of 19 health zones in the four (4) Health Districts of the city of Kinshasa.

Second level: Selection of three (3) Health Areas per Health Zone (3 x 19 = 57 Health Areas/neighbourhoods)

Third level: Three (3) streets per Health Area/neighbourhood, i.e. nine (9) per Health Area.

At the fourth level, ten households per street, i.e. thirty (30) households per Health Area/neighbourhood, ninety (90) households per Health Zone and 627 households for the entire city of Kinshasa.

2.6. Data collection techniques and tools

The following techniques were used to collect the data for this study:

- Observation of discussions during the RIA,

- Measurement of certain characteristics related to activity planning

- Structured interview based on a questionnaire. The questionnaire was designed taking into account the identification of the respondent and the elements to be sought that could help identify the reasons for resistance to COVID 19 vaccines.

2.7. List of variables

The following variables were collected:

a) Socio-demographic and economic characteristics of respondents

The socio-demographic and economic characteristics of the respondents, including the following variables of interest, were collected: sex, age, marital status, religion, level of education, household size and daily expenditure on catering in the household. The level of household income was calculated by dividing the daily household expenditure in dollars on catering by the size of the household. A household was considered to have a high level of income if it stated that it usually spent at least 1.25 dollars per person per day, and households spending less than this amount were considered to have a low level.

b) Respondents' knowledge of COVID 19:

The level of knowledge was assessed in section 2 of the questionnaire using four questions, namely: having ever heard of COVID 19; knowledge of the means of transmission of COVID 19; knowledge of the symptoms of COVID 19; knowledge of the means of prevention of COVID 19; and knowledge of toll-free numbers.

c) Risk perception and attitudes to government prevention measures

Five questions were used to measure the perception of the risk of contracting COVID 19: the risk of contracting the disease; the fear of contracting the disease; the perception of the curability of the disease and the effectiveness of prevention measures; and the acceptability of prevention measures by the community. As for attitudes, two questions were asked to measure the level of stigmatisation against COVID 19. A total score was calculated.

d) Prevention practices and the challenges encountered in implementing them

Preventive practices against COVID 19 were measured by respondents' self-declaration. The items were taken from a similar survey conducted in Iran (13) and from the barrier measures recommended by the WHO and the DRC Ministry of Health. The following items were sought: restriction of movement (five questions); prevention practices during coughing (one question); social distancing (one question); hand hygiene (one question); use of a social mask (one question); avoidance of touching the face with unwashed hands (one question); avoidance of hand-waving or kissing (one question); discussion of COVID 19 prevention with family or friends (one question).

e) Acceptability of the vaccine

We asked participants whether they would be willing to receive a vaccine to protect themselves against the coronavirus, if one were made available in the country. This variable was collected on a nominal scale (binary qualitative), coded 0 if the participant expressed a willingness to be vaccinated and 1 in the case of refusal.

f) Reason for non-acceptance of the vaccine

For participants who had not expressed a wish to receive the vaccine, additional questions were asked to investigate the reasons for this refusal.

2.8. Theoretical and ethical considerations

Ethical considerations made it possible to obtain the informed consent of respondents, ensure the confidentiality of information and guarantee the safety of the study for respondents.

The study protocol was submitted to the ethics committee for approval. Before administering the questionnaire, each investigator sought informed consent from the person to be interviewed after a brief explanation of the study's objectives. All the subjects selected were informed that participation in the study was voluntary, that they could interrupt the interview at any time and that they were not obliged to answer all the questions.

Respondent confidentiality was guaranteed as no personal

information was collected that could link the respondent to his or her data.

CONCLUSION

The Covid-19 pandemic caused a major crisis, paralysing activities in various fields throughout the world. The purpose of this study was to understand the Kinshasa population's refusal to be vaccinated against the Covid-19 pandemic and to propose a managerial strategy capable of gaining acceptance for the vaccine with the aim of eradicating this viral pandemic. The general declared objective was to contribute to the fight against COVID 19 with the aim of ending the pandemic.

In an attempt to understand the general behaviour of people who refuse to be vaccinated, the main research question revolved around the factors that explain why people in the provincial city of Kinshasa refuse the Covid-19 vaccine.

On the basis of this question, the hypotheses put forward were, in particular, that the absence of strategic and operational management does not encourage the implementation of prevention activities, that the population's resistance to vaccination is directly linked to the occurrence of MAPI, that the sidelining of community leaders at various levels has accentuated the population's refusal of vaccines, and that social networks have greatly affected the official circuit for raising the population's awareness in favour of vaccines.

To decipher all of the questions posed, we resorted to a descriptive cross-sectional analysis. The results we arrived at show that the population

of the provincial city of Kinshasa is reluctant to be vaccinated against covid

19. This resistance is due to the lack of information about vaccines against

covid 19 and more to the operational aspects of this campaign. These are

demonstrated by the low rate of vaccination against covid 19, i.e. 8.00%

since the launch of the campaign.

BIBLIOGRAPHY

I. Publications

1. EDUARD B, BATSON A., *Using immunization coverage rates for monitoring health sector performance: Measurement and interpretation issues. Human development network,* The World Bank; Washington DC. 2000; pp. 16-17.)

2. WHO, UNICEF, *Global immunization: strategic vision 2006-2015.* Geneva, 2006.

3. PROULX D., *Management des organisations publiques " théories et applications ",* 2ème Edition, Québec/Canada 2008

4. NSAMAN OLUTU O and ATSHWEL MUNTUNGI G, *Comprendre le management,* Kinshasa, CAPM, 2009.

5. PLANE J M., *Management des organisations " théories, concepts et performances,* 5ème Edition, Malakoff, Dunod, 2016.

6. MCGRATH J and BATES B., *Le petit livre des grandes théories du management,* Eyrolles, Paris, 2016.

7. RODET Ph., *Le management bienveillant,* Eyrolles bookshop, Paris, 2017.

8. ABRAHAM, YM. (2005), Du souci scolaire au sérieux managérial, ou comment devenir un HEC, enquête auprès des étudiants de HEC Paris, Cahier de recherche n°05-02, HEC Montréal, Montréal.

9. ALVAREZ, C. MAZZA, C. MUR, J. (1999), The management

publishing industry in Europe, working paper 99/4, Research division, IESE, University of Navarra, Barcelona

10. AMADO, G. ELSNER, R., *Prise de poste : les dilemmes du manager,* Paris: Village mondial, 2008.

11. ARMSTRONG, S. FUKAMI, C. (2009), The SAGE Handbook of Management Learning, Education and Development. London: SAGE Publications.

Table of Contents

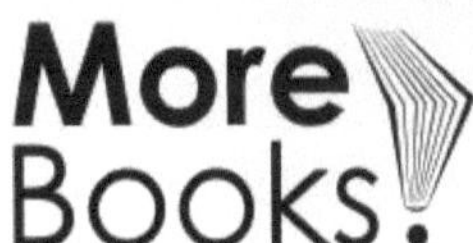
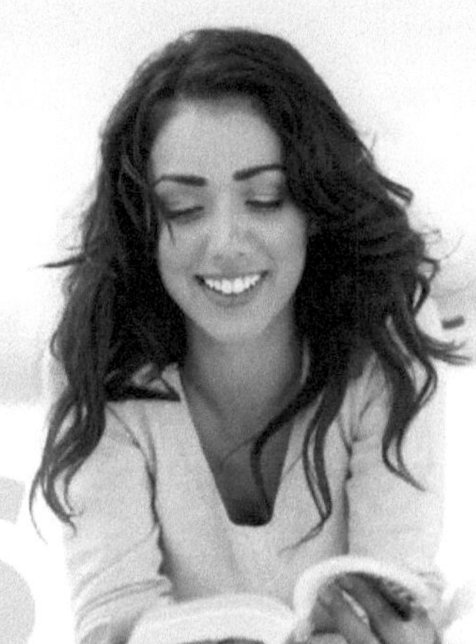

yes I want morebooks!

Buy your books fast and straightforward online - at one of world's fastest growing online book stores! Environmentally sound due to Print-on-Demand technologies.

Buy your books online at
www.morebooks.shop

Kaufen Sie Ihre Bücher schnell und unkompliziert online – auf einer der am schnellsten wachsenden Buchhandelsplattformen weltweit! Dank Print-On-Demand umwelt- und ressourcenschonend produziert.

Bücher schneller online kaufen
www.morebooks.shop

info@omniscriptum.com
www.omniscriptum.com

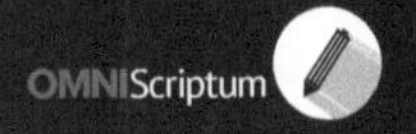

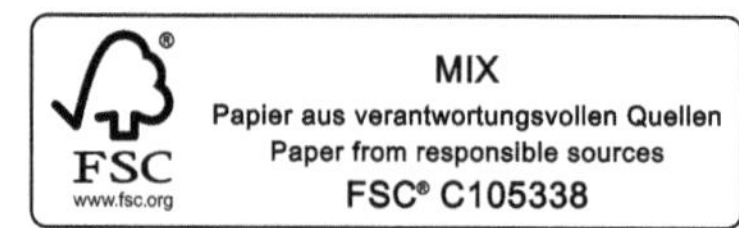